# Kindred Spirits
## Your Personal Pregnancy Journal

Tammy-Lee Ovens Watts

Author and Photographer
www.kindredspiritsphoto.com

Edited by Gordan Morash
Artwork by Erica Mills  www.warmfuzzcards.com

Note for Librarians: A cataloguing record for this book is available from Library and Archives
Canada at www.collectionscanada.ca/amicus/index-e.html
ISBN 1-4120-7245-x

*Printed in Victoria, BC, Canada. Printed on paper with minimum 30% recycled fibre. Trafford's print shop
runs on "green energy" from solar, wind and other environmentally-friendly power sources.*

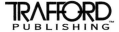

*Offices in Canada, USA, Ireland and UK*

This book was published *on-demand* in cooperation with Trafford Publishing. On-demand
publishing is a unique process and service of making a book available for retail sale to the
public taking advantage of on-demand manufacturing and Internet marketing. On-demand
publishing includes promotions, retail sales, manufacturing, order fulfilment, accounting and
collecting royalties on behalf of the author.

**Book sales for North America and international:**
Trafford Publishing, 6E–2333 Government St.,
Victoria, BC v8t 4p4 CANADA
phone 250 383 6864 (toll-free 1 888 232 4444)
fax 250 383 6804; email to orders@trafford.com
**Book sales in Europe:**
Trafford Publishing (uk) Limited, 9 Park End Street, 2nd Floor
Oxford, UK oxi 1hh UNITED KINGDOM
phone 44 (0)1865 722 113 (local rate 0845 230 9601)
facsimile 44 (0)1865 722 868; info.uk@trafford.com
**Order online at:**
trafford.com/05-2140

10 9 8 7 6 5 4 3 2

I dedicate this book to my three children
Samantha, Ryan and Keira.
Thank you for choosing me as your mother
and showing me how incredible it is
to be so deeply connected to each other.

Thank you June, whose friendship is my most precious
gift from my angels, Diana "love you,
not love you", my amazing sister Steph, my
favorite Ice Princess and my friends
Jackie (girlfriend), Irene, Margaret, Sherry,
Jocelyne, old Kate, new Kate, Siostra, Lalo
and Diane - true Kindred Spirits who have always
believed in me and constantly remind me to believe in myself.

And special thanks to my own mother who is
still with me every day, even as I write this!

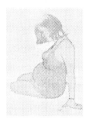

# Kindred Spirits
## Your Personal Pregnancy Journal

Every pregnant woman is beautiful inside and out, and the journey through pregnancy is one of the most amazing in life. I am fascinated with this magical season and would like to share some perceptions and insights I have learned over the years to help enhance your own personal journey through pregnancy.

I have journalled my way through three pregnancies and each time, I've learned something new about myself, about my feelings as a mother, and about my goals as a parent. Journalling is a process by which you can record your feelings about your pregnancy and the relationship you hope to share with your baby. This relationship begins in the womb and your personal pregnancy journal gives you the perfect medium through which this connection can begin.

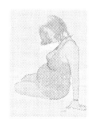

## Your Personal Pregnancy Journal

I would like to empower every pregnant woman to believe in her own power, her own intuition, and her own ability to communicate with her child and the child's guardian angels.

There are no right or wrong answers in your personal pregnancy journal. Let your pen, your mind, and your heart flow as you journal what your special pregnancy means to you. This journal has neither timelines nor an expected completion date that coincides with the birth of your baby. Use it as a guide, as a space for your thoughts, as a canvas for your doodles, as a baby name selector, a dream journal—whatever your inner self needs for expression during this time of self-reflection, personal growth and great expectancy!

*Your Personal Pregnancy Journal*

If you find deeper meaning in your own pregnancy from your journalling experience, I will feel that I have accomplished my goal.

Happy Writing & Blessings in Abundance,
Tammy-Lee Ovens Watts

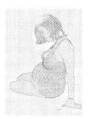

# Connecting Through Journalling

When I was about 24, I gave my mother a journal for Mother's Day. It was really cool because it had all these beautiful blank pages to be completed with prompts like: "My first day of school I remember…" and "My first best friend was…"

This was great because it was a book my mom could fill out and leave for me and future generations to enjoy. I'm not so sure my mom shared my enthusiasm.

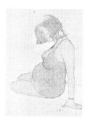

*Your Personal Pregnancy Journal*

Four years later my mom developed breast cancer and died just a few weeks after her 50th birthday.  I was given a large box of her mementoes where photos from her childhood were mixed with piano recital programs, high school report cards, wedding invitations and this Mother's Day book, still empty. Nowhere could I find a journal of any kind, a record of feelings before, during, or after my birth.

Not until I had children of my own did I realize how much I would have liked to know about my own birth and about my mom's pre-birth experiences. The only memento from my mother's pregnancy was a photograph taken two weeks before my birth.

So, should expectant moms journal only so that they leave a record of events for their future child to enjoy?

Doesn't that then create—unknowingly, of course—unwritten "should write"/"should not write" lists? Does that mean we should edit what we write and only write what we think our unborn child would like to read?

If I were fortunate enough to stumble upon a journal my mother kept, I would most definitely hope that all the sentiments, stories and dreams were true and not manufactured for my own personal benefit.

Journals are a way to bring our truths to life—now and long after ours ends.

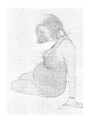

*Your Personal Pregnancy Journal*

Our journal entries need not be extravagant. Ask any child if he or she would like to hear the story of their birth and I doubt that you'd ever hear "No!" This universal interest in where we come from and how we began will never go out of style. We always will search out our stories, and your journal entries can be a way to record the ordinary and simple events that take place, as well as the "a-ha" moments you find throughout your journey.

In journalling, the only rule is that we speak our own truth. What if, after we die, someone is offended by something we've written? What if I write so much more in my first child's journal than my fifth child's? Journalling is about being in the here and now—mindfulness at its best. We must be willing to take that risk—to be fully in the present moment and journal what's in our hearts NOW, today.

Being truly present may require certain rituals that you create for yourself: a warm bath, a lighted candle, a walk in nature, whatever helps you feel more at peace (or use my Pregnancy Meditation Cards to help inspire you to find a calm space from which to write). Whichever method works for you, try to take a moment before writing so that you can fully experience your thoughts as you write them, or just doodle away if you wish!

No other structure but a date before each entry is needed. You may be a person who loves structure, so go ahead and draw lines to write on, medical notes or whatever you feel is important. There are many entries in my own pregnancy journals that include only a hand-drawn picture (an artist, I assure you, I am not) or the lyrics to a song or an ultrasound photo.

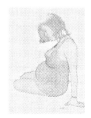

## *Your Personal Pregnancy Journal*

I admire people who journal as a regular practice and write page after page about their life. I admire them for having the personal discipline to make journalling a priority and for taking the time to really get to know themselves. For years, I have journalled and still have at least 10 half-written journals. With each new book, I vow to really finish them this time.

Journalling should not involve guilt. There are no journal police to check that everything is filled out correctly. Nor should we critique ourselves for not completing our journals. So many mothers I know have great intentions to journal throughout pregnancy and their child's early years and yet so many books lie unfinished. This journal is different. This journal is yours. *You* decide how you want it to be.

Your pregnancy journal does not have to be chronological, psychological or biological. Unlike a more traditional baby journal, there are no questions to prompt you as you write and there is no medical data to input. What really matters here is the process by which you experience the excitement and apprehensions of pregnancy. How you record the actual events is entirely up to you.

Journalling is an on-going project and you may find that this journal lasts until your child is two. Or, you may run out of space to write before you even get to your third trimester. My aim is not to write a "how-to" book on journalling. There are plenty of those on the market. My goal is to share some ideas for you to explore and show you how to personalize your own pregnancy journal.

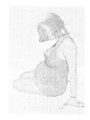

*Your Personal Pregnancy Journal*

Go ahead and read your medical and parenting books. They, too, have a place in your pregnancy journey.

Your journal is yours alone. You may or may not decide to share it with anyone, including the child you are carrying. Give yourself permission to make this your own personal journal. This is your trip—so do it your way!

Your pregnancy journal is a place where you go to escape, to dream, to hope, to ponder, to vent, to express, to communicate, to formulate, to explore and, finally, to sigh and smile. You cannot worry about what you write. You cannot edit your spelling or scribble out things that don't make sense. Everything makes sense in your journal. Your journal is your journey through a most extraordinary adventure. You are the author and your soul is the reader. May you both find each other on the pages of your pregnancy journal!

# A Spiritual Journey

As women, we focus so much on the physical health of our bodies and our babies; I was certainly no exception. While expecting my first child, I read dozens of pregnancy books and wondered about every movement, every developing organ, every craving and discomfort, and looked to the "experts" to tell me what was happening inside my own body. This seemed a perfectly normal thing to do. It helped me to learn a lot about what to expect throughout my pregnancy.

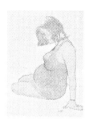

*Your Personal Pregnancy Journal*

What I could never learn from a book was how I would feel as a mother, what I would discover when I first "felt" my child's essence or how, over time, I could learn to trust my own instincts and listen to my own inner knowing as a guide to caring for my own child.

In many ways, this magical journey of pregnancy is a time of spiritual growth, and a time of spiritual and emotional preparation for the complete unknown. No woman truly knows what motherhood is like until it is fully upon her. So pregnancy is a time during which we prepare for something we really can't prepare for. What an interesting loophole in Mother Nature's plan!

The only way we can prepare for the birth of our child is to connect with him or her in our hearts and with our spirit. So how can we get to know a child who's not even born yet? Meditation, journalling, and dreams are some ways in which we can create a bond *in utero* with our child. It's amazing how attached we can become to our babies before they're even born. And this deep connection can make our relationship to our newborn even stronger when they are first in our arms.

While expecting my first child, there was a song that I often would play in the car and I would sing out loud. Sarah McLachlan's *In the Arms of an Angel*, both haunting and beautiful, may seem like an odd song to sing to my baby. For me, it was the perfect song and helped me connect with my daughter, both in and out of the womb.

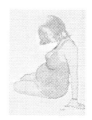

*Your Personal Pregnancy Journal*

My sister is a very talented singer. Often, throughout my mother's battle with cancer, my sister would play and sing this song. Long after my mother's death, this song played in my head and, remarkably, helped me feel more connected to both my child and my mom.

My mom had always looked forward to being a grandmother. During one of her last days, my mom confided in me how saddened she was to realize that she would not have this opportunity.

I had no immediate plans for motherhood, though I had always known that one day I would have a daughter and name her Samantha. I don't know why, but I loved this name as a little girl and it always just felt right to me as a name for the baby I would carry one day. So as my mother and I talked about this unborn child, I asked her to watch over her from Heaven one day.

And, a few days later as my mom took her last few breaths, she talked about hearing angels singing and how beautiful it sounded.

Three years later I found out that I was expecting the day before my mother's birthday. Naturally, as I carried Samantha in my womb, angels seemed to have great symbolic meaning for my pregnancy and Sarah's song so beautifully echoed that. Aside from the connections to my mom, I found such an incredible bonding experience just in the act of singing to my child *in utero*, rubbing my belly and mentally talking to my baby.

All children are connected spiritually with their parents, and singing, journalling, meditating and dreaming are just a few ways of tapping into that spiritual connection.

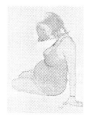

*Your Personal Pregnancy Journal*

Upon the birth of my daughter, I fully realized how much an unborn baby hears while in the womb. Whenever I played Sarah's song to my baby, there was this incredible look that would come over her face—a look of recognition and peace. This helped me feel that our connection had come full circle. In the circle of life, somehow my mother, my daughter and my sister were all connected to me through the power of music.

You will find your own symbols, songs or examples of bonding with your baby *in utero*. The important thing is to be aware that this bonding does happen and that you need only to be open to experience it.

So much research has been done on the developing baby that we now know how much these beings can absorb—auditorially, emotionally and even neurologically.  A newborn baby instinctively knows its parents' voices, the smell of its mother's milk and how to have its needs met by crying its own distinct cry (designed by nature to pull at the heartstrings of its mother).

Connecting with our baby is just a quiet moment and an instinct away. Sure, it's great to record your weight, size, circumference of the belly, and bizarre food cravings during pregnancy. For me, my first pregnancy demanded that I eat Maui Brownie Madness ice cream from Baskin Robbins almost daily, my second pregnancy inspired me to crave French fries—preferably with gravy but without was fine, too—and my third pregnancy was all about veggie subs.

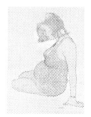

*Your Personal Pregnancy Journal*

However, the inner work we go through as we progress through this maze of giving life should not be missed. To record this inner development is to truly feel what our pregnancies mean to us.

The bonding that occurs between mother and child—kindred spirits—as a result of this inner reflection will amaze you more than anything else you can imagine!

# Connecting Through Dreams

Dreaming may be a way of connecting with our child if we are open to the mere possibility of the power of dreams.

I have always been intrigued by dreams. For years I've experienced extremely vivid and lucid dreams, and many have stayed with me for a very long time. Our dreams are our soul's way of communicating with us as the ego sleeps.

Many believe that our dreams are just snippets of our day, scattered willy-nilly throughout our brains—an instant replay of things we've seen or done.

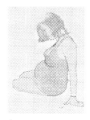

True, some dreams are mere re-enactments of things that have happened during our day, especially if we do not allow ourselves time to rest and process our day before sleeping.

Our day also enters our dreams when we watch television just before drifting off.  If, however, we allow ourselves a bedtime ritual of processing the "stuff" from the day— either through journalling, prayer, yoga, meditation, or by simply remembering each significant thing that happened and saying thanks for all our blessings—then the stage is set for the sweetest of dreams. This clears our mind and makes room for any messages that we may get as we slumber.

Rarely do we experience such vivid images, powerful emotions and strong messages as those during pregnant sleep. Plus, we're compelled to sleep more than ever as our bodies are working overtime to help our little one(s) grow.

What a rare combination: we have the opportunity *and* the enhanced awareness during this magical time of pregnancy to listen to, record and explore our dreams.

So how does the soul speak and why should we listen? Often, what we need to know about problems we are facing, decisions we are making or questions we are having is just a dream away.

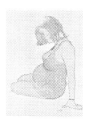

*Your Personal Pregnancy Journal*

Our Higher Self—universal energy, God, angels, whatever description feels right for you—is always trying to communicate with our conscious mind and can reach us only in the quiet gaps when we are really listening.

Quiet gaps can be deep meditation or prayer, knowing moments when we get goosebumps that signify confirmation about something, or dreams. When we need a question answered, we can ask for an answer as we drift off to sleep and wake up with a better understanding of a situation.

There are many experts lecturing on, and books written about, dreams. I believe, however, that no one is as expert as the dreamer herself. Only she knows what is represented by the symbols, colours and metaphors within her own mind.

Even if you have absolutely no interest whatsoever in dream interpretation, you might still wish to journal the significant dreams you have during your pregnancy. They will be of great interest to your child as she or he matures and you never know when the urge might overcome you to return to your dreams in the future and see what they mean.

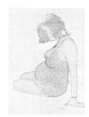

*Your Personal Pregnancy Journal*

Here is an excerpt from my first pregnancy journal:

"I had this dream at about 16 weeks…I gave
birth to you and you were a boy.  As a
baby, you could talk and we had some very
deep, spiritual talks about life…Then,
suddenly there was an invasion of some
kind and I yelled at you and dad to get in
the car as fast as possible. The streets
were being blocked off by army trucks and I
wanted to get us all out of town before
something terrible happened. Eventually
you were taken away from me and you grew
up in some kind of camp and it took until
you were 18 before I could find you. Finally I
found you and together, you and I planned
your escape. You were my 18-year-old son
Rhys who I loved with all my heart…then I
woke up!"

I haven't formally analyzed this dream and probably never will. I do, however, remember how vivid and action-packed it was and I sometimes wonder if there could be some suggestion of past life connections between my daughter and me (in this dream I had a boy, but at the time of the dream, I was carrying a girl).

It doesn't matter whether you place any importance to your dreams by seeking out their meaning, or whether you simply surrender yourself to the awe and mystery of dreams. Just by recording those that stick out in your mind the most, you'll be recording history and sharing some of the poignant memories from your pregnancy.

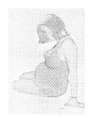

*Your Personal Pregnancy Journal*

When you wake during the night, just jot down a few notes about the dream(s) in your journal (which will, of course, be on your bedside table at all times!). In the morning, if you can still remember your dream, lie still for a little while before getting up and write more details, as much as you can remember at this time.

Rarely in a woman's life are her dreams so vivid, so strong and so jam-packed with meaning and messages. If you log your dreams in a journal only once in your life, this is the time!

# Connecting Through Intuition

Everyone has advice for the new mother. You can go absolutely crazy trying to listen to every suggestion, read every book, and make everyone else happy. There is nothing to prove and no award for being the best new mother. Everything you need to be the best mother you can be is inside yourself.

Trust yourself!

Listen to others when you need help or support, but trust your own instincts when it comes to your own child—that's why the universe gave mothers instincts!

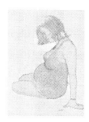

*Your Personal Pregnancy Journal*

It's not always easy to stand up for yourself and what you believe to be best for your family. When I had my first child and would nurse her to sleep at night, many more-experienced parents would warn me about the dangers of spoiling my child. When would my daughter go into her own crib? When would I start giving her a bottle or letting her cry herself to sleep alone? I realize that we all have different beliefs about the best way to put our children to sleep. I'm not suggesting that my method of having my baby in bed with me works for everyone. I'm asking you to consider what *your* thoughts are. What feels right for you?

If you try something and you get a knot in your stomach, then perhaps your body is trying to tell you something.

Well-meaning friends and family often have great advice and we can certainly save ourselves a lot of heartache by trying some of their suggestions. Just take a moment to consider each suggestion first and see if it fits for you and your child.

Let your journal be the place to explore your own personal beliefs about parenting, relationships and childhood—your own or that of your child-to-be. Give yourself the freedom to write or draw without worrying what someone else might think or what you're supposed to write. This could be good practice in learning to trust yourself as a parent, too.

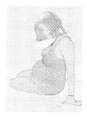

*Your Personal Pregnancy Journal*

Now is a great time to think about the things that are important to you in life, and the things you want to share with your children as they grow up. If you're open to the idea that your instincts can guide you in parenting your child, you might be able to tap into this intuition— especially now, before your baby is born.

We're forever learning new things as parents, but the core ingredient for starting out is the willingness to listen to our hearts along the way.

Intuition can show up in many ways—a physical sensation such as a knot in the stomach or goosebumps, or a sensation that can only be felt by your sixth sense.

Before I became a mom, I taught a variety of courses on personality styles. Often the question of nature vs. nurture would be asked and I always maintained that, although we are born with a particular set of preferences, we are actually socialized in the personal style we develop for life. HA! Now that I have carried three different children inside of me, I see how our children's spirit is there from the start.

That spirit, in my experience, does not change after birth. Babies are born with their personal preferences already established and, if we're tuned into our babies during the months before they're born, we may actually get clues as to what they'll be like outside the womb. Sure, given the challenges that each child will face, and our own personal parenting styles, socialization can in fact play into how a child expresses him or herself.

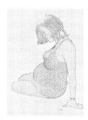

However, I now believe that we can tell a lot about our child's personality before they're even born. My second child, Ryan, is an incredibly demonstrative child who thrives on physical expressions of love—hugs, kisses, being close. In the womb, he would always "touch" back immediately after I placed my hand on my belly. Of course, all children need to feel loved but we may interpret love in different ways. Whether or not there is any scientific proof to back up my hunch, why not conduct your own study? Record any feelings or observations you have of your child before he or she is born and compare notes later to see if you were right in your guess. The point is not to get caught up in whether your gut feelings are right or wrong, they are what they are—your own personal observations about your own personal pregnancy.

And later, as a parent, your intuition will continue to play into your daily life. I still struggle with finding my own way to parent my kids. I owe it to them to do what's in my own heart and find my own way of connecting with them. Maybe my daughter would have slept through the night a lot sooner had I used a crib from the start. I'll never know what could have been.

All I know is what feels right to me. That feeling is intuition and every pregnant woman is blessed with so much of it! Let your journal help you explore what your pregnancy means to you.

Whether we know it or not, we are constantly guided by our Higher Selves.

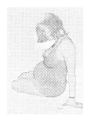

*Your Personal Pregnancy Journal*

If we are willing to listen, we'll hear whispers of our intuition when we approach a dangerous situation, when we meet someone we're meant to meet, when we stumble upon a great business idea, or when we have a personal triumph. Whatever is going on in our lives, if we listen, our intuition will guide us.

Once when my child was napping in her stroller outside in the fresh air, I heard a tap on my window. My baby was just outside the window and I was watching her very closely while I cooked and she slept. This tapping sounded exactly like someone physically knocking at the window and it came at exactly the time I had turned my back for a moment.

I knew no one was in my backyard because it was locked and I knew my child, at eight months of age, was unable to reach up and knock herself. However, when I looked outside I found that my daughter had woken up suddenly from her nap and was trying to climb out of her stroller.

I was able to run and get her before any harm could come to her. Did an angel knock on my window? Was it my late mom trying to get my attention? Maybe just a nut dropped from a passing squirrel. Whatever prompted my instincts to hear and react doesn't matter. What's important is to respond when something touches us inside.

We may or may not ever really learn to trust this inner knowing, but it is always there.

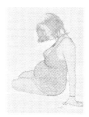

The same is true for our unborn child, with a guardian angel to help him or her through life. If we are still and open-minded, we can connect with our unborn child in a spiritual way that will leave us feeling like we've known each other our whole life.

# Connecting Through Names

A child's name is full of meaning, and finding that name can be a lengthy process. In many societies there are naming rituals, religious ceremonies and various other naming traditions. Sometimes a child will carry on the tradition of a grandparent or other family member's name. Parents-to-be will often pore over numerous baby name books and websites and, through the process of elimination, agree—or not— upon a name.

A child's name comes to parents through an intuitive process. Whether or not this is understood greatly depends on your personal view of intuition.

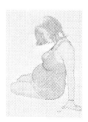

*Your Personal Pregnancy Journal*

So how does a parent's intuition play into this process? We may think of names we like and intuitively know when we've chosen the right one. Sometimes this doesn't happen until the child is born. Sometimes a name is chosen before birth only to be changed as soon as the little face emerges and the parents feel the essence of that child. I have a friend who didn't name her child for almost a week after she was born. Whatever feels right for you IS right for you.

Sometimes, our intuition lets us know after the fact that we've chosen the right name.

A girlfriend was trying to decide on a name for her baby girl. She and her husband had considered naming her after her dad. A week before the baby was born, my friend had heard the name Ruby—something about that name intrigued her. Initially, her husband wasn't intrigued at all.

To their surprise, the baby girl was born with bright red hair and so my girlfriend insisted on the name Ruby. Her husband still wasn't convinced.

Later, while driving home from the hospital, Ruby's dad hit nothing but red lights all the way home. He stopped at the store to pick up juice and for the first time noticed it was called Ruby Red Grapefruit. He was beginning to feel she was a Ruby. Finally he asked his son what names he liked. Neither my girlfriend nor her husband had told anyone about the name Ruby. Out of nowhere, the son said: "I know it's not a very common name, but I think she looks like a Ruby." How many more signs does one need?

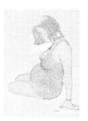

*Your Personal Pregnancy Journal*

I also received confirmation about choosing the correct name after my child was born. Having decided on the name Samantha at the age of 10, my husband felt it only fair that he name the second child. I agreed and only asked that the name be chosen by the time we found out the baby's gender on the ultrasound so that I could call the him or her in my womb by name.

I was scheduled for a C-section on November 24, 2000 and my son's name was selected long before my due date. However, on the morning of November 20, I went into labour and Ryan Gunnar (named after my husband's two favourite soccer players—Ryan Giggs and Ole Gunnar Solskjaer from Manchester United) was born a few hours later. It was not until I began writing in his baby book that I realized my son's date of birth 11-20 reflected the exact numbers on the backs of the shirts of these two soccer players. Coincidence? Maybe. Confirmation that his names were meant to be? Absolutely.

No matter how it happens, there is no question that naming your child is an extremely individual process. I suggest using this journal to help you find those quiet moments when you can reflect and get a sense of your baby's soul. She or he has feelings, hearing and intuition, even inside your womb, and you may be guided in choosing the perfect name for your little one if you're open to this possibility.

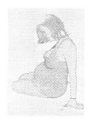

# *Your Personal Journalling Experience*

Use your journal to help you write the feelings or thoughts you have during those quiet times. Allow yourself to feel whatever comes and try not to edit or judge your feelings. Let them come and go, and write or draw whatever comes to your pen as you experience these incredible moments.

Whatever you write, whatever you feel, they're all yours. You'll enrich your pregnancy experience by allowing yourself to fully express yourself, however you choose. Enjoy and cherish this magical season.

Let this be your guide for the spiritual journey that lies ahead.

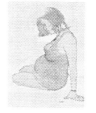

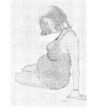

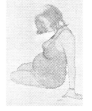

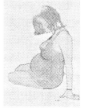

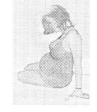

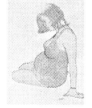

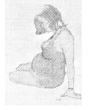

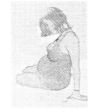

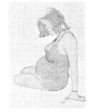

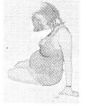

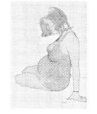

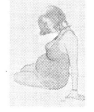

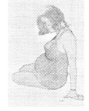

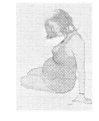

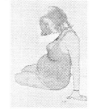

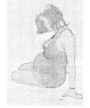

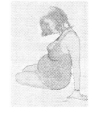

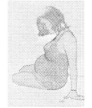

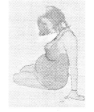

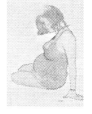

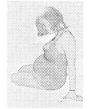

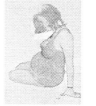

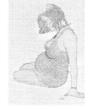

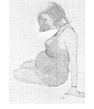

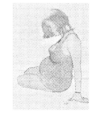

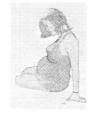

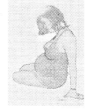

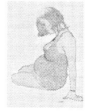

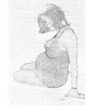

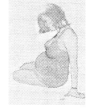

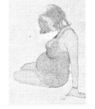

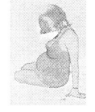

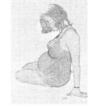

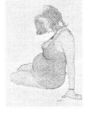

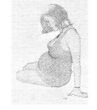

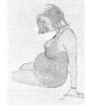

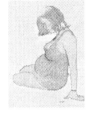

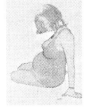

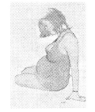

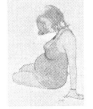

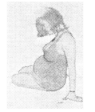

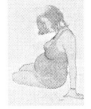

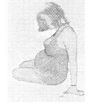

Blessings for you and your little one(s)!

# Bibliography

Chamberlain, David. <u>The Mind of Your Newborn Baby</u>. Pub Group West, North Atlantic Books, 1998, ISBN 155643264X
*"Explores new discoveries about newborns, including the phenomenon of birth memory Recognized psychologist David Chamberlain pulls together important strands from three decades of unprecedented scientific investigation to present the surprising competence of newborns, including their sensory alertness, engaging qualities of personality, and remarkable skills of communication. In the afterword he explores early memory, infant pain perception, and the life-changing power of early parent-infant bonding."*

Hilarion, writing through M.B. Cook, <u>Child Light</u>.Canada: Marcus Books, 1987, ISBN 0919951325
*"Explains the hidden side of the child-parent relationship, teaching parents how to discipline with love. use name-sounds to overcome negative traits, how to interpret the order in which teeth are cut and much more. If you've ever struggled with the problems of explaining Santa Claus and the Easter Bunny or how to teach your child the principles of the New Age, then this is the book for you."*

Jackson, Deborah. <u>Three in a Bed:  The Benefits of Sleeping with Your Baby</u>. Bloomsbury, 2003,  ISBN 0747565759
*I absolutely LOVED this book!!!  Explores the benefits of sleeping with your baby and compares western and eastern societies and traditions. Couldn't put it down until I finished it!*

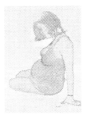

Kabat-Zinn, John and Myla.  <u>Everyday Blessings: The Inner Word of Mindful Parenting</u>. Hyperion Books, 1998, ISBN 0786883146
*An absolutely beautiful and empowering book for every parent! About learning to relax and enjoy every precious moment and parent in a more mind-ful way!*

Louden, Jennifer. <u>Pregnant Woman's Comfort Book, A Self-Nurturing Guide To Your Emotional Well-Being During Pregnancy and Early Motherhood</u>. Harpercollins, Little Brown,  2001  ISBN 0060776722
*With the wit, humor, and style that have made her Comfort Book series so popular, mother Jennifer Louden brings her wisdom to the sometimes wonderful, sometimes overwhelming world of pregnancy. From the blissful moments to the panic attacks, Louden guides women through the precarious emotional terrain of pregnancy and early motherhood*

Martina, Irene and associates. <u>Dream Masters</u>. To be published in 2006.
www.irenemartina.com
*Thank you, Irene, my dream teacher and friend. You are a very wise and generous soul.*

Sears, William, M.D. and Martha Sears.  <u>The Attachment Parenting Book</u>.
Little Brown. 2001. ISBN 0316778095
Thank you Dr. Sears!  You helped me feel empowered as a mother and you were way ahead of your time!!!

ISBN 141207245-X